# Experiments Upon Heat. By Major-General Sir Benjamin Thompson, Knt. F.R.S. in a Letter to Sir Joseph Banks, Bart. P.R.S. From the Philosophical Transactions

EXPERIMENTS UPON HEAT.

BY

MAJOR-GENERAL SIR BENJAMIN THOMPSON, Knt.
F. R. S.

IN A LETTER TO

SIR JOSEPH BANKS, Bart. P.R.S.

FROM THE

PHILOSOPHICAL TRANSACTIONS

EXPERIMENTS UPON HEAT.

Read before the ROYAL SOCIETY, *January* 19, 1792.

DEAR SIR, *Munich, June,* 1787.

Since my last communication upon the subject of HEAT, which the Royal Society have done me the honour to publish in their Transactions, I have made some further progress in the investigation of that most interesting subject, of which I propose to give you an account in this letter.

The confining and directing of heat are objects of such vast importance in the œconomy of human life, that I have been induced to confine my researches chiefly to those points, conceiving that very great advantages to mankind could not fail to be derived from the discovery of any new facts relative to these operations

If the laws of the communication of heat from one body to another were known, measures might be taken with certainty, in all cases, for confining it, and directing its operations, and this would not only be productive of great œconomy in the articles of fuel and clothing, but would likewise greatly increase the comforts and conveniencies of life; objects of which the philosopher should never lose sight

The route which I have followed in this inquiry is that which I thought bid fairest to lead to useful discoveries. Without embarrassing myself with any particular theory, I have formed to myself a plan of experimental investigation, which I conceived would conduct me to the knowledge of certain facts, of which we are now ignorant, or very imperfectly informed, and with which it is of consequence that we should be made acquainted.

The first great object which I had in view in this inquiry was to ascertain, if possible, the cause of the warmth of certain bodies; or the circumstances upon which their power of confining heat depends. This, in other words, is no other than to determine the cause of the conducting and non-conducting power of bodies.

To this end I began by determining by actual experiment the relative conducting powers of various bodies of very different natures, both fluids and solids, of some of which experiments I have already given an account in the Paper above mentioned, which is published in the Transactions of the Royal Society for the year 1786, I shall now, taking up the matter where I left it, give you the continuation of the history of my researches.

Having discovered that the Torricellian vacuum is a much worse conductor of heat than common air, and having ascertained the relative conducting powers of air, of water, and of mercury, under different circumstances, I proceeded to examine the conducting powers of various solid bodies, and particularly of such substances as are commonly made use of for clothing.

The method of making these experiments was as follows: a mercurial thermometer,[*] whose bulb was about $\frac{55}{100}$ of an inch

---

[*] See Phil. Trans. Vol. LXXVI. Tab. VI. Fig. 4.

Experiments upon Heat.

in diameter, and its tube, about 10 inches in length, was suspended in the axis of a cylindrical glass tube, about $\frac{3}{4}$ of an inch in diameter, ending with a globe $1\frac{6}{10}$ inch in diameter, in such a manner that the centre of the bulb of the thermometer occupied the centre of the globe; and the space between the internal surface of the globe and the surface of the bulb of the thermometer being filled with the substance whose conducting power was to be determined, the instrument was heated in boiling water, and afterwards being plunged into a freezing mixture of pounded ice and water, the times of cooling were observed, and noted down.

The tube of the thermometer was divided at every tenth degree from 0°, or the point of freezing, to 80°, that of boiling water, and these divisions being marked upon the tube with the point of a diamond, and the cylindrical tube being left empty, the height of the mercury in the tube of the thermometer was seen through it.

The thermometer was confined in its place by means of a stopple of cork, about $1\frac{1}{2}$ inch long, fitted to the mouth of the cylindrical tube, through the centre of which the end of the tube of the thermometer passed, and in which it was cemented.

The operation of introducing into the globe the substances whose conducting powers are to be determined, is performed in the following manner; the thermometer being taken out of the cylindrical tube, about two-thirds of the substance which is to be the subject of the experiment are introduced into the globe; after which, the bulb of the thermometer is introduced a few inches into the cylinder; and, after it, the remainder of the substance being placed round about the tube of the thermometer; and, lastly, the thermometer being introduced farther into the tube, and being brought into its proper place, that part of the substance which, being introduced last, remains in the cylindrical tube above the bulb of the thermometer, is pushed down into the globe, and placed equally round the bulb of the thermometer by means of a brass wire which is passed through holes made for that purpose in the stopple closing the end of the cylindrical tube.

As this instrument is calculated merely for measuring the passage of heat in the substance whose conducting power is examined, I shall give it the name of *passage-thermometer*, and I shall apply the same appellation to all other instruments constructed upon the same principles, and for the same use, which I may in future have occasion to mention, and as this instrument has been so particularly described, both here, and in my former Paper upon the subject of heat, in speaking of any others of the same kind in future it will not be necessary to enter into such minute details. I shall, therefore, only mention their *sizes*, or the diameters of their bulbs, the diameters of their globes, the diameters of their cylinders, and the lengths and divisions of their tubes, taking it for granted that this will be quite sufficient to give a clear idea of the instrument.

In most of my former experiments, in order to ascertain the conducting power of any body, the body being introduced into the globe of the passage-thermometer, the instrument was cooled to the temperature of freezing water, after which, being taken out of the ice water, it was plunged suddenly into boiling water, and the times of heating from ten to ten degrees were observed and noted; and I said that these times were as the conducting power of the body inversely; but in the experiments of which I am now about to give an account, I have in general reversed the operation; that is to say, instead of observing the times of heating, I have first heated the body in boiling water, and then plunging it into a mixture of pounded ice and ice-cold water, I have noted the times taken up in cooling.

I have preferred this last method to the former, not only on account of the greater ease and convenience with which a thermometer, plunged into a mixture of water, may be observed, than when placed in a vessel of boiling water, and surrounded by hot steam, but also on account of the greater accuracy of the experiment, the heat of boiling water varying with the variations of the pressure of the atmosphere consequently the experiments made upon different days will have different results, and of course, strictly speaking, cannot be compared together; but the temperature of pounded ice and water is ever the same, and of course the results of the experiments are uniform.

In heating the thermometer, I did not in general bring it to the temperature of the boiling water, as this temperature, as I have just observed, is variable; but when the mercury had attained the $75°$ of its scale, I immediately took it out of the boiling water, and plunged it into the ice and water; or, which I take to be still more accurate, suffering the mercury to rise a degree or two above $75°$, and then taking it out of the boiling water, I held it over the vessel containing the pounded ice and water, ready to plunge it into that mixture the moment the mercury, descending, passes the $75°$.

Having a watch at my ear which beat half seconds (which I counted), I noted the time of the passage of the mercury over the divisions of the thermometer, marking 70° and every tenth degree from it, descending, to 10° of the scale. I continued the cooling to 0°, or the temperature of the ice and water, in very few instances, as this took up much time, and was attended with no particular advantage, the determination of the times taken up in cooling 60 degrees of REAUMUR's scale, that is to say, from 70° to 10°, being quite sufficient to ascertain the conducting power of any body whatever.

During the time of cooling in ice and water, the thermometer was constantly moved about in this mixture from one place to another; and there was always so much pounded ice mixed with the water, that the ice appeared above the surface of the water; the vessel, which was a large earthen jar, being first quite filled with pounded ice, and the water being afterwards poured upon it, and fresh quantities of pounded ice being added as the occasion required.

Having described the apparatus made use of in these experiments, and the manner of performing the different operations, I shall now proceed to give an account of the experiments themselves.

My first attempt was to discover the relative conducting powers of such substances as are commonly made use of for clothing; accordingly, having procured a quantity of *raw silk*, as spun by the worm, *sheep's wool, cotton wool, linen* in the form of the finest lint, being the scrapings of very fine Irish linen, the finest part of the *fur of the beaver*, separated from the skin, and from the long hair, the finest part of the *fur of a white Russian hare*, and *Eider down*; I introduced successively 16 grains in weight of each of these substances into the globe of the passage-thermometer, and placing it carefully

Experiments upon Heat.

and equally round the bulb of the thermometer, I heated the thermometer in boiling water, as before described, and taking it out of the boiling water, plunged it into pounded ice and water, and observed the times of cooling.

But as the interstices of these bodies thus placed in the globe were filled with air, I first made the experiment with air alone, and took the result of that experiment, as a standard by which to compare all the others; the results of three experiments with air were as follows:

	The bulb of the thermometer surrounded by air.			
Heat lost	Exp No 1 Time elapsed	Exp No 2 Time elapsed	Heat acquired.	Exp No 3 Time elapsed
70°	—	—	10°	—
60°	38″	38″	20°	39″
50°	46	46	30°	43
40°	59	59	40°	53
30°	80	79	50°	67
20°	122	122	60°	96
10°	231	230	70°	175
Total times	576	574	—	473

The following table shows the results of the experiments, with the various substances therein mentioned:

Heat lost.	Air.	Raw silk, 16 grs.	Sheep's wool, 16 grs.	Cotton wool, 16 grs.	Fine lint, 16 grs.	Beavers fur, 16 grs.	Hares fur, 16 grs.	Eider down, 16 grs.
	Exp. 1	Exp. 4	Exp 5	Exp 6	Exp 7.	Exp 8	Exp 9	Exp 10
70°	—	—	—	—	—	—	—	—
60°	38″	94″	79″	83″	80″	99″	97″	98″
50°	46	110	95	95	93	116	117	116
40°	59	133	118	117	115	153	144	146
30°	80	185	162	152	150	185	193	192
20°	122	273	238	221	218	265	270	268
10°	231	489	426	378	376	478	494	485
Total times.	576	1284	1118	1046	1032	1296	1315	1305

Now the *warmth* of a body, or its power to confine heat, being as its power of resisting the passage of heat through it (which I shall call its *non-conducting power*), and the time taken up by any body in cooling, which is surrounded by any medium through which the heat is obliged to pass, being, *cæteris paribus*, as the resistance which the medium opposes to the passage of the heat, it appears that the *warmth* of the bodies mentioned in the foregoing table are as the times of cooling; the *conducting powers* being inversely as those times, as I have formerly shown.

From the results of the foregoing experiments it appears, that of the seven different substances made use of, hares fur and Eider down were the warmest; after these came beavers fur; raw silk; sheep's wool; cotton wool; and lastly, lint, or the scrapings of fine linen; but I acknowledge that the

Experiments upon Heat.

differences in the warmth of these substances were much less than I expected to have found them.

Suspecting that this might arise from the volumes or solid contents of the substances being different (though their weights were the same), arising from the difference of their specific gravities; and as it was not easy to determine the specific gravities of these substances with accuracy, in order to see how far any known difference in the volume or quantity of the same substance, confined always in the same space, would add to, or diminish the time of cooling, or the apparent warmth of the covering, I made the three following experiments.

In the first, the bulb of the thermometer was surrounded by 16 grains of Eider down; in the second by 32 grains; and in the third by 64 grains, and in all these experiments the substance was made to occupy exactly the same space, viz. the whole internal capacity of the glass globe, in the centre of which the bulb of the thermometer was placed; consequently the thickness of the covering of the thermometer remained the same, while its density was varied in proportion to the numbers 1, 2, and 4.

The results of these experiments were as follow:

The following table shows the results of the experiments, with the various substances therein mentioned:

Heat lost	Air. Exp 1	Raw silk, 16 grs. Exp 4.	Sheep's wool, 16 grs. Exp 5	Cotton wool, 16 grs. Exp 6	Fine lint, 16 grs. Exp. 7	Beavers fur, 16 grs. Exp 8	Hares fur, 16 grs. Exp 9	Eider down, 16 grs. Exp 10
70°	—	—	—	—	—	—	—	—
60°	38″	94″	79″	83″	80″	99″	97″	98″
50°	46	110	95	95	93	116	117	116
40°	59	133	118	117	115	153	144	146
30°	80	185	162	152	150	185	193	192
20°	122	273	238	221	218	265	270	268
10°	231	489	426	378	376	478	494	485
Total times	576	1284	1118	1046	1032	1296	1315	1305

Now the *warmth* of a body, or its power to confine heat, being as its power of resisting the passage of heat through it (which I shall call its *non-conducting power*), and the time taken up by any body in cooling, which is surrounded by any medium through which the heat is obliged to pass, being, *cæteris paribus*, as the resistance which the medium opposes to the passage of the heat, it appears that the *warmth* of the bodies mentioned in the foregoing table are as the times of cooling; the *conducting powers* being inversely as those times, as I have formerly shown.

From the results of the foregoing experiments it appears, that of the seven different substances made use of, hares fur and Eider down were the warmest; after these came beavers fur; raw silk; sheep's wool; cotton wool; and lastly, lint, or the scrapings of fine linen; but I acknowledge that the differences in the warmth of these substances were much less than I expected to have found them.

Suspecting that this might arise from the volumes or solid contents of the substances being different (though their weights were the same), arising from the difference of their specific gravities; and as it was not easy to determine the specific gravities of these substances with accuracy, in order to see how far any known difference in the volume or quantity of the same substance, confined always in the same space, would add to, or diminish the time of cooling, or the apparent warmth of the covering, I made the three following experiments

In the first, the bulb of the thermometer was surrounded by 16 grains of Eider down; in the second by 32 grains; and in the third by 64 grains; and in all these experiments the substance was made to occupy exactly the same space, viz. the whole internal capacity of the glass globe, in the centre of which the bulb of the thermometer was placed; consequently the thickness of the covering of the thermometer remained the same, while its density was varied in proportion to the numbers 1, 2, and 4.

The results of these experiments were as follow :

The bulb of the thermometer being surrounded by Eider down.			
Heat lost	16 grains.	32 grains.	64 grains.
	(Exp No. 11)	(Exp. No 12)	(Exp No 13)
70°	—	—	—
60°	97″	111″	112″
50°	117	128	130
40°	145	157	165
30°	192	207	224
20°	267	304	326
10°	486	565	658
Total times	1304	1472	1615

Without stopping at present to draw any particular conclusions from the results of these experiments, I shall proceed to give an account of some others, which will afford us a little further insight into the nature of some of the circumstances upon which the warmth of covering depends.

Finding, by the last experiments, that the density of the covering added so considerably to the warmth of it, its thickness remaining the same, I was now desirous of discovering how far the internal structure of it contributed to render it more or less pervious to heat, its thickness and quantity of matter remaining the same. By internal structure, I mean the disposition of the parts of the substance which forms the covering; thus they may be extremely divided, or very fine, as raw silk as spun by the worms, and they may be equally distributed through the whole space they occupy; or they may be coarser,

Experiments upon Heat.

or in larger masses, with larger interstices, as the ravelings of cloth, or cuttings of threads.

If heat passed *through* the substances made use of for covering, and if the warmth of the covering depended solely upon the difficulty which the heat meets with in its passage through the substances, *or solid parts,* of which they are composed, in that case, the warmth of covering would be always, *cæteris paribus,* as the quantity of materials of which it is composed, but that this is not the case, the following, as well as the foregoing experiments clearly evince.

Having, in the experiment N° 4, ascertained the warmth of 16 grains of raw silk, I now repeated the experiment with the same quantity, or weight, of the ravelings of white taffety, and afterwards with a like quantity of common sewing silk, cut into lengths of about two inches.

The following table shows the results of these three experiments:

Heat lost.	Raw silk, 16 grs	Ravelings of taffety, 16 grs	Sewing silk cut into lengths, 16 grs
	Exp 4	Exp 14.	Exp 15
70°	—	—	—
60°	94″	90″	67″
50°	110	106	79
40°	133	128	99
30°	185	172	135
20°	273	246	195
10°	489	427	342
Total times.	1284	1169	917

Here, notwithstanding that the quantities of the silk were the same in the three experiments, and though in each of them it was made to occupy the same space, yet the warmth of the coverings which were formed were very different, owing to the different disposition of the material.

The raw silk was very fine, and was very equally distributed through the space it occupied, and it formed a warm covering

The ravelings of taffety were also fine, but not so fine as the raw silk, and of course the interstices between its threads were greater, and it was less warm; but the cuttings of sewing silk were very coarse, and consequently it was very unequally distributed in the space in which it was confined; and it made a very bad covering for confining heat.

It is clear from the results of the five last experiments, that the air which occupies the interstices of bodies, made use of for covering, acts a very important part in the operation of confining heat; yet I shall postpone the examination of that circumstance till I shall have given an account of several other experiments, which, I think, will throw still more light upon that subject.

But, before I go any farther, I will give an account of three experiments which I made, or rather the same experiment which I repeated three times the same day, in order to see how far experiments made according to the method here described, may be depended on, as being regular in their results.

The glass globe of the passage-thermometer being filled with 16 grains of cotton-wool, the instrument was heated and cooled three times successively, when the times of cooling were observed as follows:

Heat lost	Exp 16	Exp 17	Exp 18
70°	—	—	—
60°	82″	84″	83″
50°	96	95	95
40°	118	117	116
30°	152	153	151
20°	221	221	220
10°	380	377	377
Total times	1049	1047	1042

The difference of the times of cooling in these three experiments were extremely small; but regular as these experiments appear to have been in their results, they were not more so than the other experiments made in the same way, many of which were repeated two or three times, though, for the sake of brevity, I have put them down as single experiments.

But to proceed in the account of my investigations relative to the causes of the warmth of warm clothing. Having found that the fineness and equal distribution of a body or substance made use of to form a covering to confine heat, contributes so much to the warmth of the covering, I was desirous, in the next place to see the effect of condensing the covering, its quantity of matter remaining the same, but its thickness being diminished in proportion to the increase of its density.

The experiment I made for this purpose was as follows:— I took 16 grains of common sewing silk, neither very fine nor very coarse, and winding it about the bulb of the thermometer in such a manner that it entirely covered it, and was as nearly as possible of the same thickness in every part, I replaced the thermometer in its cylinder and globe, and heating it in boiling water, cooled it in ice and water, as in the foregoing experiments. The results of the experiment were as may be seen in the following table; and in order that it may be compared with those made with the same quantity of silk differently disposed of, I have placed those experiments by the side of it:

Heat lost	Raw silk, 16 grs	Fine ravelings of taffety, 16 grs.	Sewing silk, cut into lengths, 16 grs	Sewing silk, 16 grs wound round the bulb of the thermometer
	Exp No 4	Exp No 14	Exp. No 15	Exp No 19
70°	—	—	—	—
60°	94″	90″	67″	46″
50°	110	106	79	62
40°	133	128	99	85
30°	185	172	135	121
20°	273	246	195	191
10°	489	427	342	399
Total times	1284	1169	917	904

It is not a little remarkable, that, though the covering formed of sewing silk wound round the bulb of the thermometer in the 19th experiment, appeared to have so little power of confining the heat when the instrument was very hot, or when it was first plunged into the ice and water, yet afterwards, when the heat of the thermometer approached much nearer to that of the surrounding medium, its power of confining the heat which remained in the bulb of the thermometer appeared to be even greater than that of the silk in the experiment N° 15, the time of cooling from 20° to 10° being in the one 399″, and

Experiments upon Heat.

in the other 342″. The same appearance was observed in the following experiments, in which the bulb of the thermometer was surrounded by threads of *wool*, of *cotton*, and of *linen*, or *flax*, wound round it, in the like manner as the sewing silk was wound round it in the last experiment.

The following table shows the results of these experiments, with the threads of various kinds; and that they may the more easily be compared with those made with the same quantity of the same substances in a different form, I have placed the accounts of these experiments by the side of each other. I have also added the account of an experiment, in which 16 grains of fine linen cloth were wrapped round the bulb of the thermometer, going round it nine times, and being bound together at the top and bottom of it, so as completely to cover it.

Heat lost	*Sheeps wool*, 16 grains, surrounding the bulb of the thermometer.	*Woollen thread*, 16 grains, wound round the bulb of the thermometer	*Cotton wool*, 16 grains, surrounding the bulb of the thermometer	*Cotton thread*, 16 grains, wound round the bulb of the thermometer	*Lint*, 16 grains, surrounding the bulb of the thermometer	*Linen thread*, 16 grains, wound round the bulb of the thermometer	*Linen cloth*, 16 grains, wrapped round the bulb of the thermometer
	Exp 5	Exp 20	Exp 6	Exp 21	Exp 7	Exp 22	Exp 23
70°	—	—	—	—	—	—	—
60°	79″	46″	83″	45″	80″	46″	42″
50°	95	63	95	60	93	62	56
40°	118	89	117	83	115	83	74
30°	162	126	152	115	150	117	108
20°	238	200	221	179	218	180	168
10°	426	410	378	370	376	385	338
Total times	1118	934	1046	852	1032	873	783

That thread wound light round the bulb of the thermometer should form a covering less warm than the same quantity of wool, or other raw materials of which the thread is made, surrounding the bulb of the thermometer in a more loose manner, and consequently occupying a greater space, is no more than what I expected, from the idea I had formed of the causes of the warmth of covering; but I confefs I was much surprised to find that there is so great a difference in the relative warmth of these two coverings, when they are employed to confine great degrees of heat, and when the heat they confine is much less in proportion to the temperature of the surrounding medium. This difference was very remarkable, in the experiments with sheep's wool, and with woolen thread, the warmth of the covering formed of 16 grains of the former, was to that formed of 16 grains of the latter, when the bulb of the thermometer was heated to 70° and cooled to 60°, as 79 to 46 (the surrounding medium being at 0°); but afterwards, when the thermometer had only fallen from 20° to 10° of heat, the warmth of the wool was to that of the woolen thread only as 4,26 to 4,10; and in the experiments with lint, and with linen thread, when the heat was much abated, the covering of the thread appeared to be even warmer than that of the lint, though in the beginning of the experiments, when the heat was much greater, the lint was warmer than the thread, in the proportion of 80 to 46.

From hence it should seem that a covering may, under certain circumstances, be very good for confining small degrees of warmth, which would be but very indifferent when made use of for confining a more intense heat, and *vice versa*. This, I believe, is a new fact; and, I think the knowledge of it may lead to further discoveries relative to the causes of the warmth of coverings, or the manner in which heat makes its passage through them. But I forbear to enlarge upon this subject, till I shall have given an account of several other experiments, which I think throw more light upon it, and which will consequently render the investigation easier and more satisfactory.

With a view to determine how far the power which certain bodies appear to possess of confining heat, when made use of as covering, depends upon the natures of those bodies, considered as chymical substances, or upon the chymical principles of which they are composed, I made the following experiments.

As charcoal is supposed to be composed almost entirely of phlogiston, I thought that, if that principle was the cause either of the conducting power, or the non-conducting power of the bodies which contain it, I should discover it by making the experiment with charcoal, as I had done with various other bodies. Accordingly, having filled the globe of the passage-thermometer with 176 grains of that substance in very fine powder (it having been pounded in a mortar, and sifted through a fine sieve), the bulb of the thermometer being surrounded by this powder, the instrument was heated in boiling water, and being afterwards plunged into a mixture of pounded ice and water, the times of cooling were observed as mentioned in the following table. I afterwards repeated the experiment with lampblack, and with very pure, and very dry wood ashes; the results of which experiments were as under mentioned:

The bulb of the thermometer surrounded by			
Heat lost	176 grains of fine powder of charcoal.	176 grains of fine powder of charcoal	195 grains of lampblack	307 grains of pure dry wood ashes
	Exp No 24	Exp No 25	Exp No. 26	Exp No 27.
70°	—	—	—	—
60°	79″	91″	124″	96″
50°	95	91	118	92
40°	100	109	134	107
30°	139	133	164	136
20°	196	192	237	185
10°	331	321	394	311
Total times	940	937	1171	927

The experiment, N° 25, was simply a repetition of that numbered 24, and was made immediately after it; but, in moving the thermometer about in the former experiment, the powder of charcoal which filled the globe was shaken a little together, and to this circumstance I attribute the difference in the results of the two experiments.

In the experiments with lampblack and with wood ashes, the times taken up in cooling from 70° to 60° were greater than those employed in cooling from 60° to 50°; this most probably arose from the considerable quantity of heat contained by these substances, which was first to be disposed of, before they could receive and communicate to the surrounding medium that which was contained by the bulb of the thermometer.

Experiments upon Heat.

The next experiment I made was with *semen lycopodii*, commonly called witch-meal, a substance which possesses very extraordinary properties. It is almost impossible to wet it; a quantity of it strewed upon the surface of a basin of water, not only swims upon the water without being wet, but it prevents other bodies from being wet which are plunged into the water through it; so that a piece of money, or other solid body, may be taken from the bottom of the basin by the naked hand, without wetting the hand; which is one of the tricks commonly shown by the jugglers in the country: this meal covers the hand, and descending along with it to the bottom of the basin, defends it from the water. This substance has the appearance of an exceeding fine, light, and very moveable yellow powder, and it is very inflammable; so much so, that being blown out of a quill into the flame of a candle, it flashes like gunpowder, and it is made use of in this manner in our theatres for imitating lightning.

Conceiving that there must have been a strong attraction between this substance and air, and suspecting, from some circumstances attending some of the foregoing experiments, that the warmth of a covering depends not merely upon the fineness of the substance of which the covering is formed, and the disposition of its parts, but that it arises in some measure from a certain attraction between the substance and the air which fills its interstices, I thought that an experiment with *semen lycopodii* might possibly throw some light upon this matter; and in this opinion I was not altogether mistaken, as will appear by the results of the three following experiments.

Heat lost	Cooled Exp No 28	Cooled Exp No 29	Heat acquired	Heated Exp No 30
The bulb of the therm. surrounded by 256 grs. of *semen lycopodii*.					

Heat lost	Cooled Exp No 28	Cooled Exp No 29	Heat acquired	Heated Exp No 30
70°	—	—	0°	—
60°	146"	157"	10°	230"
50°	162	160	20°	68
40°	175	170	30°	63
30°	209	203	40°	76
20°	284	288	50°	121
10°	502	513	60°	316
—	—	—	70°	1585
Total times	1478	1491	—	2459

In the last experiment (N° 30) the result of which was so very extraordinary, the instrument was cooled to 0° in thawing ice, after which it was plunged suddenly into boiling water, where it remained till the inclosed thermometer had acquired the heat of 70°, which took up no less than 2456 seconds, or above 40 minutes; and it had remained in the boiling water full a minute and an half before the mercury in the thermometer shewed the least sign of rising. Having at length been put into motion, it rose very rapidly 40 or 50 degrees, after which its motion gradually abating became so slow, that it took up 1585 seconds, or something more than 26 minutes in rising from 60° to 70°, though the temperature of the medium in which it was placed during the whole of this time was very nearly 80°; the mercury in the barometer standing but little short of 27 Paris inches.

Experiments upon Heat.

All the different substances which I had yet made use of in these experiments for surrounding or covering the bulb of the thermometer, fluids excepted, had, in a greater, or in a less degree confined the heat, or prevented its passing into or out of the thermometer so rapidly as it would have done, had there been nothing but air in the glass globe, in the centre of which the bulb of the thermometer was suspended. But the great question is, how, or in what manner, they produced this effect?

And first, it was not in consequence of their own non-conducting powers, simply considered; for, if instead of being only bad conductors of heat, we suppose them to have been totally impervious to heat, their volumes or solid contents were so exceedingly small in proportion to the capacity of the globe in which they were placed, that, had they had no effect whatever upon the air filling their interstices, that air would have been sufficient to have conducted all the heat communicated, in less time than was actually taken up in the experiment.

The diameter of the globe being 1,6 inches, its contents amounted to 2,14466 cubic inches; and the contents of the bulb of the thermometer being only 0,08711 of a cubic inch, (its diameter being 0,55 of an inch) the space between the bulb of the thermometer and the internal surface of the globe amounted to $2,14466 - 0,08711 = 2,05755$ cubic inches; the whole of which space was occupied by the substances by which the bulb of the thermometer was surrounded in the experiments in question.

But though these substances occupied this space, they were far from filling it; by much the greater part of it being filled by the air which occupied the interstices of the substances in question. In the experiment N° 4, this space was occupied by 16 grains of raw silk; and as the specific gravity of raw silk is to that of water as 1734 to 1000, the volume of this silk was equal to the volume of 9,4422 grains of water; and as 1 cubic inch of water weighs 253,185 grains, its volume was equal to $\frac{9,4422}{253,1850} = 0,037294$ of a cubic inch; and, as the space it occupied amounted to 2,05755 cubic inches, it appears that the silk filled no more than about $\frac{1}{55}$ part of the space in which it was confined, the rest of that space being filled with air.

In the experiment N° 1, when the space between the bulb of the thermometer and the glass globe, in the centre of which it was confined, was filled with nothing but air, the time taken up by the thermometer in cooling from 70° to 10° was 576 seconds; but in the experiment N° 4, when this same space was filled with 54 parts air, and 1 part raw silk, the time of cooling was 1284 seconds.

Now, supposing that the silk had been totally incapable of conducting any heat at all, if we suppose, at the same time, that it had no power to prevent the air remaining in the globe from conducting it, in that case its presence in the globe could only have prolonged the time of cooling in proportion to the quantity of the air it had displaced to the quantity remaining, that is to say, as 1 is to 54, or a little more than 10 seconds. But the time of cooling was actually prolonged 708 seconds, (for in the experiment N° 1, it was 576 seconds, and in the experiment N° 4, it was 1284 seconds, as has just been observed); and this shows, that the silk not only did not conduct the heat itself, but that it prevented the air by which its interstices were filled from conducting it; or, at least, it greatly weakened its power of conducting it.

The next question which arises is, how air can be prevented from conducting heat? and this necessarily involves another, which is, how does air conduct heat?

If air conducted heat, as it is probable that the metals and water, and all other solid bodies and unelastic fluids conduct it, that is to say, if its particles remaining in their places, the heat passed from one particle to another, through the whole mass, as there is no reason to suppose that the propagation of heat is necessarily in right lines, I cannot conceive how the interposition of so small a quantity of any solid body as $\frac{1}{55}$ part of the volume of the air, could have effected so remarkable a diminution of the conducting power of the air, as appeared in the experiment (N° 4) with raw silk, above mentioned.

If air and water conducted heat in the same *manner*, it is more than probable that their conducting powers might be impaired by the same means; but when I made the experiment with water, by filling the glass globe, in the centre of which the bulb of the thermometer was suspended, with that fluid, and afterwards varied the experiment, by adding 16 grains of raw silk to the water, I did not find that the conducting power of the water was sensibly impaired by the presence of the silk.

But we have just seen that the same silk, mixed with an equal volume of air, diminished its conducting power in a very remarkable degree; consequently, there is great reason to conclude that water and air conduct heat in a *different manner*.

But the following experiment, I think, puts the matter beyond all doubt.

It is well known, that the power which air possesses of

holding water in solution is augmented by heat, and diminished by cold, and that, if hot air is saturated with water, and if this air is afterwards cooled, a part of its water is necessarily deposed. I took a cylindrical bottle of very clear transparent glass, about 8 inches in diameter, and 12 inches high, with a short and narrow neck, and suspending a small piece of linen rag, moderately wet, in the middle of it, I plunged it into a large vessel of water, warmed to about 100° of Fahrenheit's thermometer, where I suffered it to remain till the contained air was not only warm, but thoroughly saturated with the moisture which it attracted from the linen rag, the mouth of the bulb being well stopped up during this time with a good cork; this being done, I removed the cork for a moment, to take away the linen rag, and stopping up the bottle again immediately, I took it out of the warm water, and plunged it into a large cylindrical jar, about 12 inches in diameter, and 16 inches high, containing just so much ice-cold water, that, when the bottle was plunged into it, and quite covered by it, the jar was quite full.

As the jar was of very fine transparent glass, as well as the bottle, and as the cold water contained in the jar was perfectly clear, I could see what passed in the bottle most distinctly; and having taken care to place the jar upon a table near the window, in a very favourable light, I set myself to observe the appearances which should take place, with all that anxious expectation which a conviction that the result of the experiment must be decisive, naturally inspired.

I was certain, that the air contained in the bottle could not part with its heat, without at the same time, that is to say, *at the same moment*, and *in the same place*, parting with a proportion

Experiments upon Heat.

of its water; if therefore, the heat penetrated the mass of air from the centre to the surface, or *passed through it* from particle to particle, in the same manner as it is probable that it passes through water, and all other unelastic fluids, by far the greatest part of the air contained in the bottle would part with its heat, when *not actually in contact with the glass,* and a proportional part of its water being let fall at the same time, and in the *same place,* would necessarily descend in the form of rain; and, though this rain might be too fine to be visible in its descent, yet I was sure I should find it at the bottom of the bottle, if not in visible drops of water, yet in that kind of cloudy covering which cold glass acquires from a contact with hot steam or watery vapour.

But if the particles of air, instead of communicating their heat from one to another, from the centre to the surface of the bottle, each in its turn, and for itself, came to the surface of the bottle, and there deposited its heat, and its water, I concluded that the cloudiness occasioned by this deposit of water would appear all over the bottle, or, at least, not more of it at the bottom than at the sides, but rather less; and this I found to be the case in fact.

The cloudiness first made its appearance upon the sides of the bottle, near the top of it; and from thence it gradually spread itself downwards, till, growing fainter as it descended lower, it was hardly visible at the distance of half an inch from the bottom of the bottle; and upon the bottom itself, which was nearly flat, there was scarcely the smallest appearance of cloudiness.

These appearances, I think, are easy to be accounted for. The air immediately in contact with the glass being cooled, and having deposited a part of its water upon the surface of the glass, at the same time that it communicates to it its heat, slides downwards by the sides of the bottle in consequence of its increased specific gravity, and, taking its place at the bottom of the bottle, forces the whole mass of hot air upwards ; which, in its turn coming to the sides of the bottle, *there* deposites its heat and its water, and afterwards bending its course downwards, this circulation is continued till all the air in the bottle has acquired the exact temperature of the water in the jar.

From hence it is clear why the first appearance of condensed vapour is near the top of the bottle, as also why the greatest collection of vapour is in that part, and that so very small a quantity of it is found nearer the bottom of the bottle.

This experiment confirmed me in an opinion which I had for some time entertained, that, though the particles of air individually, or each for itself, are capable of receiving and *transporting* heat, yet air in a quiescent state, or as a fluid whose parts are at rest with respect to each other, is not capable of conducting it, or giving it a passage ; in short, that heat is incapable of *passing through a mass of air*, penetrating from one particle of it to another, and that it is to this circumstance that its non-conducting power is principally owing.

It is also to this circumstance, in a great measure, that it is owing that its non-conducting power, or its apparent warmth when employed as a covering for confining heat, is so remarkably increased upon being mixed with a small quantity of any very fine, light, solid substance, such as the raw silk, fur, Eider down, &c. in the foregoing experiments : for as I have already observed, though these substances, in the very small quantities in which they were made use of, could hardly have prevented, in any considerable degree, the air from conducting, or giving a *passage* to the heat, had it been capable of passing through it, yet they might very much impede it in the operation of transporting it.

But there is another circumstance which it is necessary to take into the account, and that is the attraction which subsists between air and the bodies above mentioned, and other like substances, constituting natural and artificial clothing. For, though the incapacity of air to give a passage to heat in the manner solid bodies and non-elastic fluids permit it to pass through them, may enable us to account for its warmth under certain circumstances, yet the bare admission of this principle does not seem to be sufficient to account for the very extraordinary degrees of warmth which we find in furs and in feathers, and in various other kinds of natural and artificial clothing, nor even that which we find in snow; for if we suppose the particles of air to be at liberty to *carry off* the heat which these bodies are meant to confine, without any other obstruction or hinderance than that arising from their *vis inertiæ*, or the force necessary to put them in motion, it seems probable that the succession of fresh particles of cold air, and the consequent loss of heat, would be much more rapid than we find it to be in fact.

That an attraction, and a very strong one, actually subsists between the particles of air, and the fine hair or furs of beasts, the feathers of birds, wool, &c. appears by the obstinacy with which these substances retain the air which adheres to them, even when immersed in water, and put under the receiver of an air-pump; and that this attraction is essential to the warmth of these bodies, I think is very easy to be demonstrated.

In furs, for instance, the attraction between the particles of air, and the fine hairs in which it is concealed, being greater than the increased elasticity, or repulsion of those particles with regard to each other, arising from the heat communicated to them by the animal body, the air in the fur, though heated, is not easily displaced; and this coat of confined air is the real barrier which defends the animal body from the external cold. This air cannot *carry off* the heat of the animal, because it is itself confined, by its attraction to the hair or fur; and it transmits it with great difficulty, if it transmits at all, as has been abundantly shewn by the foregoing experiments.

Hence it appears why those furs which are the finest, longest, and thickest, are likewise the warmest; and how the furs of the beaver, of the otter, and of other like quadrupeds which live much in water, and the feathers of water-fowls, are able to confine the heat of those animals in winter, notwithstanding the extreme coldness and great conducting power of the water in which they swim. The attraction between these substances, and the air which occupies their interstices, is so great, that this air is not dislodged even by the contact of water, but remaining in its place, it defends the body of the animal at the same time from being wet, and from being robbed of its heat by the surrounding cold fluid; and it is possible that the pressure of this fluid upon the covering of air confined in the interstices of the fur, or feathers, may at the same time increase its warmth, or non-conducting power, in such a manner that the animal may not, in fact, lose more heat when in water, than when in air: for we have seen by the foregoing experiments, that, under certain circumstances, the warmth of a covering is increased, by bringing its component parts nearer together, or by increasing its density even at the expence of its thickness. But this point will be further investigated hereafter.

Bears, wolves, foxes, hares, and other like quadrupeds, inhabitants of cold countries, which do not often take the water, have their fur much thicker upon their backs than upon their bellies. The heated air occupying the interstices of the hairs of the animal tending naturally to rise upwards, in consequence of its increased elasticity, would escape with much greater ease from the backs of quadrupeds than from their bellies, had not Providence wisely guarded against this evil by increasing the obstructions in those parts, which entangle it and confine it to the body of the animal. And this, I think, amounts almost to a proof of the principles assumed relative to the manner in which heat is carried off by air, and the causes of the non-conducting power of air, or its apparent warmth, when, being combined with other bodies, it acts as a covering for confining heat.

The snows which cover the surface of the earth in winter, in high latitudes, are doubtless designed by an all-provident Creator as a garment to defend it against the piercing winds from the polar regions, which prevail during the cold season.

These winds, notwithstanding the vast tracts of continent over which they blow, retain their sharpness as long as the ground they pass over is covered with snow; and it is not till, meeting with the ocean, they acquire, from a contact with its waters, the heat which the snows prevent their acquiring from the earth, that the edge of their coldness is taken off, and they gradually die away and are lost.

The winds are always found to be much colder when the ground is covered with snow than when it is bare, and this extraordinary coldness is vulgarly supposed to be communicated to the air by the snow; but this is an erroneous opinion; for these winds are in general much colder than the snow itself.

They retain their coldness, because the snow prevents them from being warmed at the expence of the earth; and this is a striking proof of the use of the snows in preserving the heat of the earth during the winter, in cold latitudes.

It is remarkable that these winds seldom blow from the poles directly towards the equator, but from the land towards the sea. Upon the eastern coast of North America the cold winds come from the north-west; but upon the western coast of Europe, they blow from the north-east.

That they should blow towards those parts where they can most easily acquire the heat they are in search of, is not extraordinary; and that they should gradually cease and die away, upon being warmed by a contact with the waters of the ocean, is likewise agreeable to the nature and causes of their motion; and if I might be allowed a conjecture respecting the principal use of the seas, or the reason why the proportion of water upon the surface of our globe is so great, compared to that of the land, it is to maintain a more equal temperature in the different climates, by heating or cooling the winds which at certain periods blow from the great continents.

That cold winds actually grow much milder upon passing over the sea, and that hot winds are refreshed by a contact with its waters, is very certain; and it is equally certain that the winds from the ocean are, in all climates, much more temperate than those which blow from the land.

In the islands of Great Britain and Ireland, there is not the least doubt but the great mildness of the climate is entirely owing to their separation from the neighbouring continent by so large a tract of sea; and in all similar situations, in every part of the globe, similar causes are found to produce similar effects.

The cold north-west winds, which prevail upon the coast of North America during the winter, seldom extend above 100 leagues from the shore, and they are always found to be less violent, and less piercing, as they are further from the land.

These periodical winds from the continents of Europe and North America prevail most towards the end of the month of February, and in the month of March; and I conceive that they contribute very essentially towards bringing on an early spring, and a fruitful summer, particularly when they are very violent in the month of March, and if at that time the ground is well covered with snow. The whole atmosphere of the polar regions being, as it were, transported into the ocean by these winds, is there warmed and saturated with water: and, a great accumulation of air upon the sea being the necessary consequence of the long continuance of these cold winds from the shore, upon their ceasing the warm breezes from the sea necessarily commence, and, spreading themselves upon the land far and wide, assist the returning sun in dismantling the earth of the remains of her winter garment, and in bringing forward into life all the manifold beauties of the new-born year.

This warmed air which comes in from the sea, having acquired its heat from a contact with the ocean, is, of course, saturated with water; and hence the warm showers of April and May, so necessary to a fruitful season.

The ocean may be considered as the great reservoir and equalizer of heat; and its benign influences in preserving a proper temperature in the atmosphere operate in all seasons and in all climates.

The parching winds from the land under the torrid zone are cooled by a contact with its waters, and, in return, the breezes from the sea, which at certain hours of the day, come in to the shores in almost all hot countries, bring with them refreshment, and, as it were, new life and vigour both to the animal and vegetable creation, fainting and melting under the excessive heats of a burning sun. What a vast tract of country, now the most fertile upon the face of the globe, would be absolutely barren and uninhabitable on account of the excessive heat, were it not for these refreshing sea-breezes? And is it not more than probable, that the extremes of heat and of cold in the different seasons in the temperate and frigid zones would be quite intolerable, were it not for the influence of the ocean in preserving an equability of temperature?

And to these purposes the ocean is wonderfully well adapted not only on account of the great power of water to absorb heat, and the vast depth and extent of the different seas (which are such that one summer or one winter could hardly be supposed to have any sensible effect in heating or cooling this enormous mass); but also on account of the continual circulation which is carried on in the ocean itself, by means of the currents which prevail in it. The waters under the torrid zone being carried by these currents towards the polar regions, are there cooled by a contact with the cold winds, and, having thus communicated their heat to these inhospitable regions, return towards the equator, carrying with them refreshment for those parching climates.

The wisdom and goodness of Providence have often been called in question with regard to the distribution of land and water upon the surface of our globe, the vast extent of the ocean having been considered as a proof of the little regard that has been paid to man in this distribution. But, the more light we acquire relative to the real constitution of things, and the various uses of the different parts of the visible creation, the less we shall be disposed to indulge ourselves in such frivolous criticisms.

www.ingramcontent.com/pod-product-compliance
Lightning Source LLC
LaVergne TN
LVHW021823280425
809759LV00035B/101